From Zero to Ten and Back Again:
Living with Chronic Pain.

Michelle Flint

Illustrated by Jonathan Short

ISBN: 978-1983554599

DEDICATION

To my husband Derek, daughters Sara-Jane and Kayleigh, grandchildren, Leighton and Lilly, my shining lights in the darkness.

ACKNOWLEDGMENTS

I would like to express my gratitude to the many people who have supported me in the writing of this book. Many have offered comments, assisted with editing, talked through things with me and generally offered words of wisdom and support. In particular I would like to thank my husband Derek for putting up with me as I regurgitated information and clarified chronologies, Ian, for the many car rides to work and for being a listening ear, and Penny for your support and encouragement which enabled me to put pen to paper.

Special thanks must go to some additional people for supporting me through my uncertain journey with injury, rehabilitation and chronic pain: Dr Conrad Engelbrecht, Braemar Pain Clinic: Hamish Deverall, Orthopaedic Spine Surgeon; Paul Holloway and the team at TBI Health Hamilton; Niamh O'Connor, QRS Hamilton; the team at Focused Physiotherapy, Te Awamutu; Craig Newlands, Body Performance Clinic, Cambridge; Sandhya Fernandez, Clinical Psychologist; Greg Dodunski, Total Rehab Plus; Annemarie Janssens, Focus on Potential; Accident Compensation Corporation (ACC), New Zealand; River Radiology Hamilton.

And….anyone else who I may inadvertently have missed.

Finally, I would like to thank Lorimer Moseley, David Butler and Russ Harris for helping me through to the other side with their amazing books; 'Explain Pain' and 'The Happiness Trap'. Thank you gentlemen for being kind enough to allow me to quote your work in my book.

CONTENTS

Introduction

I wanted to write this book for anyone experiencing chronic pain either personally or indirectly, as a family member, health professional or support person. This is my story, a person with no medical background or prior experience of persistent pain. Someone who never really needed pain medication, other than the occasional headache remedy, and someone whose life changed dramatically because of an injury, which eventually led to chronic pain.

This account of my journey with pain, 'From Zero to Ten and Back Again', is an honest account of what happened to me and how I changed my thinking, my diet, my exercise routine and my approach to getting on top of the roller coaster ride with chronic pain. If you are living with persistent pain, you might not know the reason why. Maybe an old injury has healed but the pain remains, either the same or worse than before. Maybe it is months, or even years after your injury or surgery, but the pain has never left. Either way, persistent pain can have significant effects on your everyday life, and even worse, on your mental health.

My story will take you through the difficulties I experience while living with on-going pain. Chronic pain, for me, was not an easy diagnosis to accept. It was not easy to change my thinking and let go of the safety net of doctors, physiotherapists and psychologists that worked so closely with me for many months and years. This story will outline the approach I took to getting better and how it changed my thinking and my life almost back to where I was before the pain began and, to large extent, gave me a better and healthier quality of life afterwards.

How it all began

Not being a sporty person meant that injury and pain for gain was not something that sat comfortably with me. I could never see the pleasure in diving for a ball and having several people dive on top of me, or risking pain and injury in any sport really. Therefore, I didn't do it! Being a trained musician, I was well aware of the hours required to perfect a skill or technique in order to perform at my best. However, trumpet players, of which I am one, don't risk too much damage perfecting their art, luckily. This often makes me wonder whether or not people who are used to, or expect injury and pain, people who push themselves to attain the perfect shape, attain faster speeds to beat their personal best, cope with pain better than us non sporty mortals?

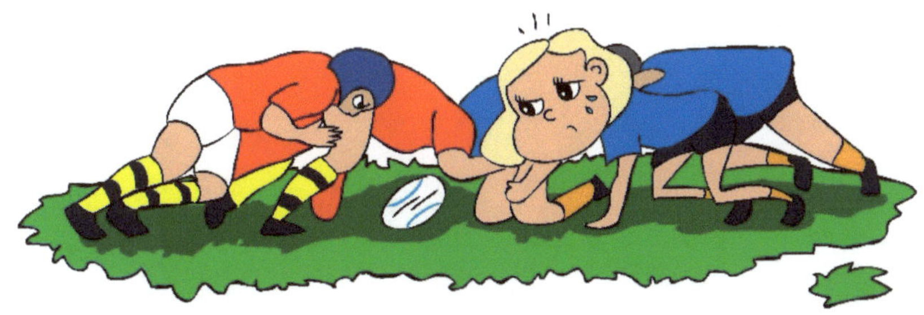

We live in a world of get up and get moving, which is great, but I know there are many people, like me, who just don't. Not necessarily because they don't want to, but quite possibly because it is not something they are used to, make time in their schedule for, or enjoy doing. Therefore when an injury happens, to the likes of us, it comes as quite a shock, and it certainly did to me.

My injury happened in July 2014, after lifting a table. My daughter and I had decided to move our very heavy, almost brand new, dining table to a different location in the house. To re-site the table, we needed to get it through a narrow hallway that was far too small and narrow for the table to fit through. Therefore, I made a very irrational decision, which I have regretted ever since, to tip the table on its side and then slide it through the narrow gap. We began this foolish task and up-ended the table. Our plan was going quite well when suddenly, there was a very loud snap and the table leg, on the opposite side to where I was lifting, broke. This left the two of us holding on for dear life to one side of the table and the other side balancing on one leg, which I was certain would snap too. I panicked, more because I was thinking about my husband and his reaction when he came home from work, and I made the impulsive decision to send my daughter to the other side of the table to try to push the broken leg back in place and to distribute the load. It hadn't dawned on me, at the time, that this very manoeuvre would leave me alone to take the full weight of the table. Anyway, to cut a very long story short, the said event resulted in the prolapse of my L4/L5/S1 spinal discs, the lowest vertebrae in the lumbar spine.

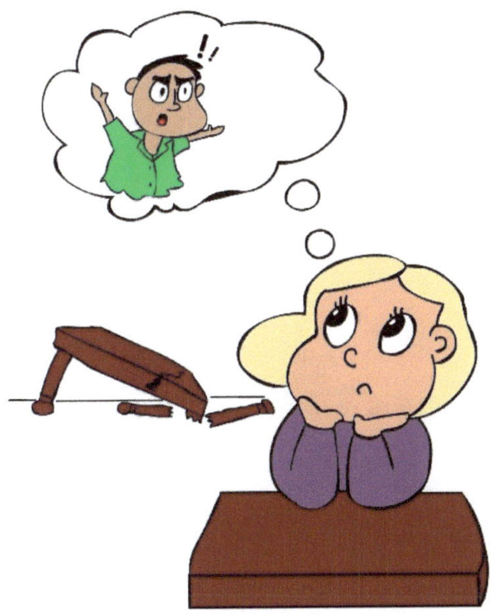

I didn't realise the damage I had done initially and it took a few weeks before the pain in my right leg became severe enough for me to visit a physiotherapist. At the time, I had no idea that the pain I was experiencing in my leg, in fact, came from prolapsed discs in my back. The pain was predominantly in my right leg and buttock and I thought that I had just pulled a muscle. Not really understanding bodily mechanisms and not used to injury, I was definitely not prepared for what was to come.

In the months following my injury I had an epidural injection to relieve the pain, and several physiotherapy sessions. When neither seemed to be helping, a Magnetic Resonance Image

(MRI) scan was scheduled. The resulting image, of a very large protruding disc came as quite a shock to me.

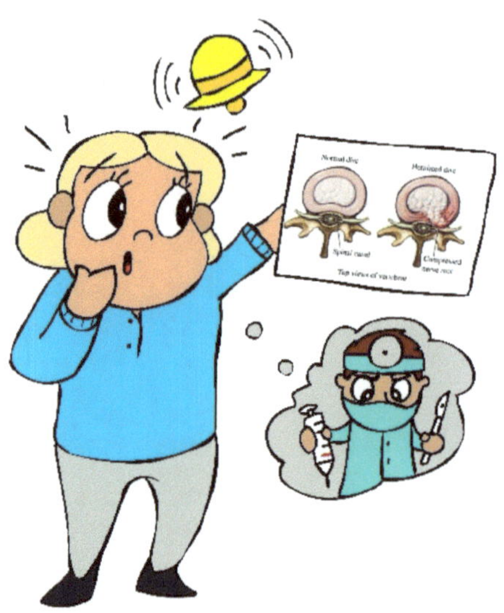

Worse still, came the devastating news that I would need surgery to remove the herniation, a discectomy, the surgical removal of the whole or a part of an intervertebral disc. What, shock, horror, no! I may as well tell you now that surgery and especially a general anaesthetic were on my biggest ever phobia list! Yes, I am a coward, there you go, I've admitted it. And, being a 21st century internet surfer, I Googled spinal discectomy surgery. Big mistake! Intense fear, alarm bells, alarm bells, what the heck? Note to self, avoid Google surfing medical conditions at all times!

I was faced with spinal surgery which, after Googling it, scared the living daylights out of me. On top of this I had had a fear of general anesthetic, after many visits to the dentist as a child.

Without giving away my age, I grew up in a time when general anaesthetics were administered in a dental surgery, with very little precaution by today's standards. As a young child I was taken to see the dentist, usually wearing my best Sunday dress, as a visit <u>out</u> was a visit <u>out</u> and you always got dressed up. Anyway, I would sit in the waiting room with the gas heater blaring away, waiting for my name to be called. Immediately, my toothache went! 'I'm cured', I would yell. 'No need to take my tooth out'. No good though; help was not at hand to rescue me from the dreaded dentist's chair. Slowly, I would ascend the steps to my inescapable doom and was greeted by my dentist who, by the way, had the blackest misshapen teeth I had ever seen, or to this day have ever seen, in my life.

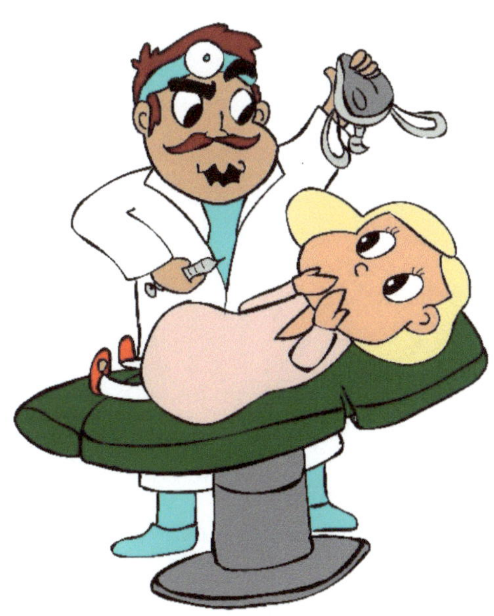

I slowly advanced to the chair! Next was the dreadful sound of the trolley containing the gas bottle being wheeled towards me. To add insult to injury the dentist would ask me which mask I would like. The one that fits just over your nose or the one that covers your nose and mouth? As if it mattered, I didn't want either. Therefore, the unavoidable happened and, to make things worse, I was held down in the chair, screaming until I drifted off to wherever you drift off to, breathing in that terrible gas. I didn't want to breathe it in, but at the same time I had to because the only way forward was to do it and get it over with.

So, that's why I don't, to this day, like the idea of having a general anaesthetic. By the way, the Sunday best white dress that I wore on my last young childhood visit to the dentist was, I believe, thrown away after that since the blood stains never came out, despite several soaks in Vim, Jazz and Ajax.

Pain Scale

I can't ever remember having pain badly enough to warrant me relating it in terms of pain intensity via a pain scale, prior to my spinal injury. You will almost certainly know the one I'm talking about, where you rate your pain from zero to ten, where zero means no pain at all and ten is the worst pain possible, to help us to decide where our pain fits and how severe it is.

By December 2014 the pain for me was becoming quite bad and, after being asked to rate my pain on numerous occasions, I decided to make my own pain scale, based on the Brosh pain scale, to fit in with my quirky sense of humour:

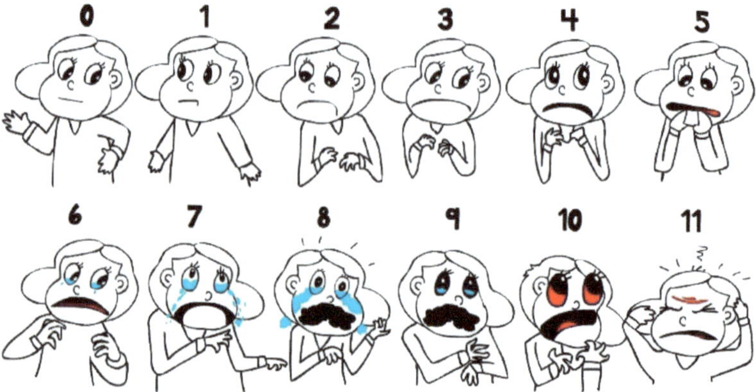

1: Did something just bite me?
2: OK...something did bite me.
3: Not happy, I don't like this.
4: This really hurts and I want it to go away.
5: What did I do to deserve this?
6: This is really not good and I am very scared.
7: This is getting disturbing and my eyes are leaking badly.
8: Oh God, I think I am dying...I really need help badly.
9: Death is imminent, I see a tunnel and bright light.
10: What, I'm still alive...how can that be?
11: Off the scale, stop asking me about my pain there are not enough numbers.

The Dreaded Surgery

As Christmas 2014 approached, nothing I did relieved the pain, whether it was medication or physiotherapy. I knew the unavoidable surgery was imminent and, by then, I had almost welcomed it, as I needed the pain to stop. The up-and-coming Christmas season made it very difficult for me to get an appointment with a spinal surgeon to discuss surgery. I carried on but, by then, the pain for me was becoming extremely bad at 'seven out of ten'. Nothing I did relieved it and I remember having excruciating spasms in my right leg that felt like huge electric shocks.

As I awaited a hospital appointment, my pain intensity definitely began to increase and I honestly did think that I must have something serious going on. On the eve of my visit to the Emergency Room, I had sat up rather too quickly when an intense 'ten out of ten' pain shot down my right leg. After that, I became numb from the waist down, on my right side. I'm not really sure how I got through that night, but the following morning I couldn't move without screaming in pain. We dialled 111, the paramedics arrived and somehow, they managed to transfer me into an ambulance as the pain had left the scale at 'eleven out of ten' and was too bad for numbers.

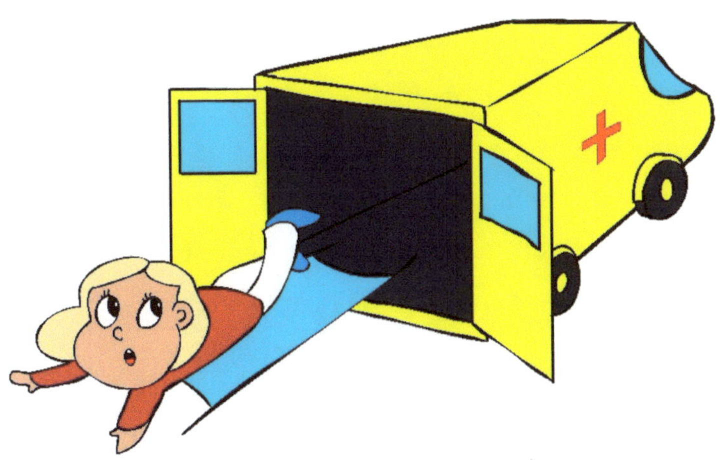

In hospital I was very scared and didn't understand what was happening to me, I was petrified and inconsolable. I remember saying that I'd given birth to two children and never thought that I could be in any worse pain. Within a couple of days my bladder stopped working and I had to face the inevitable surgery and general anaesthetic that I so dreaded. My worst nightmares came to fruition all at once

So that's how it all began for me, and I strongly believe that my fear of returning to this helpless, frightening, petrifying state of out-of-control 'eleven out of ten pain', a pain too bad for numbers, led me on a journey into the unknown realm of chronic pain.

Surgery and afterwards

I had my first surgery in December 2014. I can't really remember too much about the dreaded pre-surgery anaesthetic experience, other than it was definitely not like my childhood memories of visits to the dentist and I was very well looked after. Post-surgery, the pain was not too bad as then I only had the soreness from the surgery wound. Some areas of numbness and weakness remained in my right leg and foot, and still do today. I was discharged with strict instructions not to bend, twist or lift for around six weeks, and at least up until my first post-operative consultation.

As Christmas was approaching, I was quite emotional post-surgery. Christmas to our family is quite a big thing. Therefore, not being able to prepare in the usual way was hard and quite emotional for me. However, I stuck to my discharge instructions to the letter with no bending, twisting or lifting. Christmas dinner consisted of sliced beef on bread rolls with gravy, not our usual spread, but I was able to feel that I had at least contributed in some way.

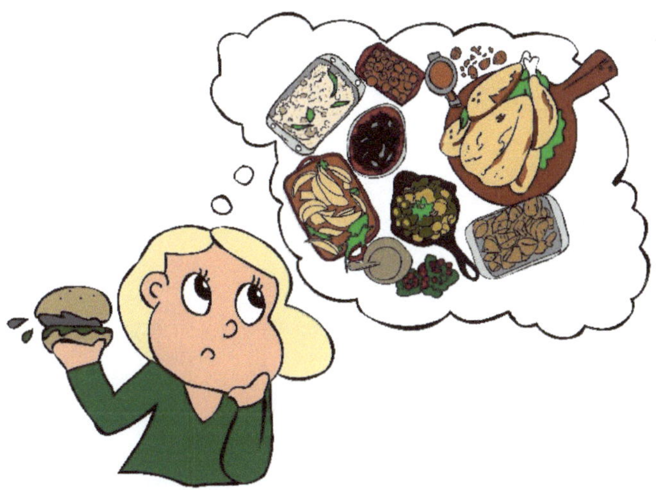

I remember feeling quite useless, as the list of things I wasn't supposed to do far out-weighed the list of things that I could. However, the end was in sight and I looked forward to a family holiday in Napier early in January.

Our holiday journey to Napier was interesting, to say the least, and we had a four-hour drive ahead of us. I think the journey there took us most of the day, as we stopped on many occasions so that I could get out, stretch my legs and move around. I remember feeling good and well on the road to recovery. I am a teacher and surgery happened at the end of the school year, so I was feeling positive that I would be almost back to normal by the start of the new school year. I just needed the go-ahead from my surgeon at my post-operative consultation.

Post-operative consultation

In January 2015 I had my post-operative consultation. I had a few questions ready for the surgeon, mainly about my return to work, which was only one week away, and the possibility of some physiotherapy. I was in a happy place and felt that I had done really well with my post-operative care.

My daughter accompanied me to the appointment and we sat and waited for the surgeon to come into the treatment room. I remember a nurse coming in and dropping my notes on the desk beside me. Then in walked a doctor whom I didn't recognise. I was about to tell him that he was in the wrong room, when he sat down and told me that he was standing in for my surgeon who was away on holiday.

Now, I don't know about you, but I see doctors as pinnacles of society. I put them on pedestals and have a great deal of admiration for what they do.

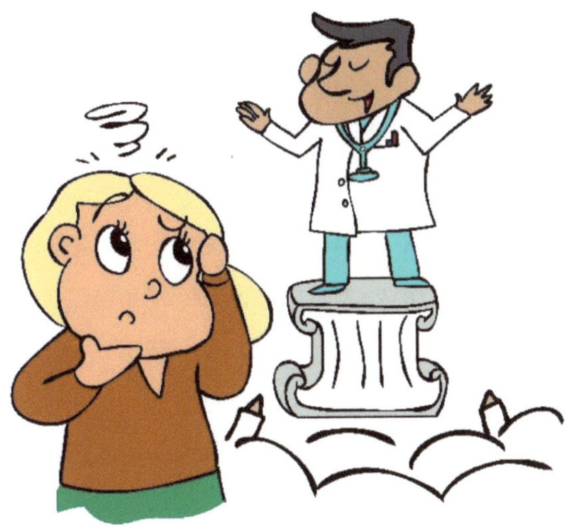

I wholeheartedly trust everything doctors say and certainly don't question it. You see, I'm from a generation where you respect a doctor's opinion and you take what they say as gospel. Therefore, if instructed to do something I certainly wouldn't query it. The doctor asked me to bend down and touch my toes. I was a little shocked and confused and did question this, only because I had spent many weeks avoiding this manoeuvre at all cost. Anyway, the instruction was repeated and I was told that I should continue to bend so that he could see how far down I could go. The doctor continued to say that this movement should be done regularly at home in the shower, gradually increasing the bend. I stood in the treatment room and did what was asked of me.

I can't really describe the pain that followed, other than I almost passed out. I remember having tears in my eyes and feeling sick to my stomach. I was then asked to lie down on a couch and the doctor proceeded to do a straight leg raise test, a passive test, which is used to evaluate a lumbar L4-S1 nerve impingement. The test is done while the patient lies on their back. The leg is raised slowly while the ankle is grasped. The lift is supposed to be done until the patient complains of pain or until maximum flexion has been reached, usually between a sixty to one-hundred-and-twenty degree angle. A positive straight leg test for sciatica is reported when pain is felt at a forty degree angle or less. The straight leg test began with my left leg, which was fine. The doctor then went to my right leg and flexed my leg to forty degrees. I complained of severe pain but he continued to raise my leg further. Without going into too much detail, the inevitable happened and a disc had prolapsed once again.

The outcome of all this was a treatment injury, leading to an investigation by the Health and Disability Commission, and this is still ongoing today.

And so it began

Trust is not something that you get back easily and my confidence in a health practitioner had been severely compromised. I don't know whether this was the trigger to my chronic pain, or whether it was the months of recovery from the second surgery that followed. Either way, my persistent pain has remained with me from then on.

In the May of 2015 I had my second surgery, a further discectomy but this time with a laminectomy, the removal of the back part of the vertebra that covers the spinal cord. This is done to create space and it relieves pressure on the nerves. The second injury, surgery and rehabilitation led to an extended period of seven months off work for me. This period was the longest and most challenging seven months of my life. As an active relaxer, having to go through rest and gradual rehabilitation, once again, was a nightmare.

I remember dreading going to physiotherapy because I was certain that I would be asked to do something that would cause me further harm. I was afraid to move and be active in case I risked additional damage to my back. I was told time and time again that the pain I was feeling, when exercising, would lead to positive results. However, it was hard to listen, as my brain was telling me to stop exercising and moving and to avoid it as much as possible. In actual fact, contrary to this fear, movement is essential to healing. I needed to stay active with short, frequent, gentle exercise.

During this time, I tried to keep positive and, with the help of my physiotherapist, set myself goals, the first of which was a six kilometer charity walk, something I had never done in my life before. When I considered enrolling in the event I was only able to walk three to four hundred meters without severe pain. Somehow, post-surgery for the second time, my recovery was very slow and pain became a normal part of everyday life. I almost anticipated the pain on a daily basis and looked for it if it wasn't there.

Additionally, I struggled to believe that I wouldn't prolapse a disc again. In my mind, every trip, slip, stumble or fall meant serious danger. To me my back was fragile, weak and in danger of harm. I listened to every warning sign in my brain that suggested threat and I acted on it. Any pain that reminded me of my pre-surgery discomfort was distressing. Reassurance from my physiotherapist did little to help as I was convinced that I was susceptible to further injury.

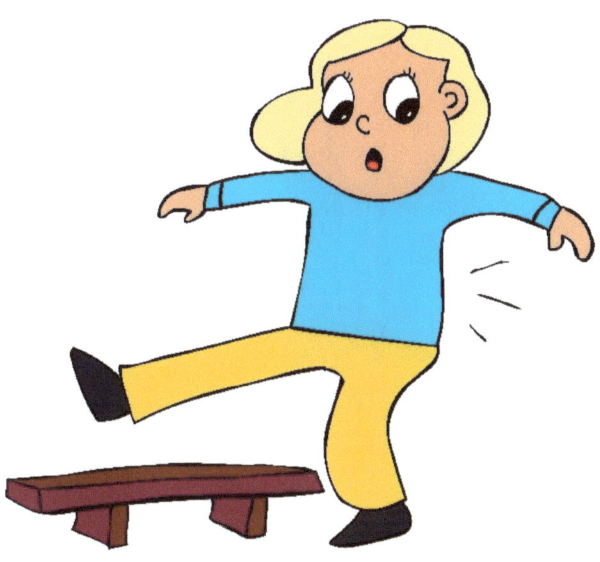

This was a dreadful state to be in, my right foot was very weak and, as I trained for the charity walk, I experienced a number of trips and falls. Every time this happened, I went into panic mode. I would re-live and visualise the surgeries, the pain, the upset and struggle. What I didn't realise, at the time, was that I was starting to re-wire my pain receptors to over exaggerate every event that would possibly put my back at risk of serious harm.

When this happened I would cut back on the exercising and revert to sitting, or lying on the couch. I found that when I had times of inactivity, my range of motion was lost and I became very stiff, even getting out of a chair became difficult. I knew from this that I had to remain active, as movement promotes healthy blood circulation, bringing oxygen to the healing site. I pushed myself to walk and walk a little further every day. I completed a six kilometer walk and proudly displayed the medal.

My wound had healed, the physiotherapy continued, my medication was increased and slowly I became fitter. In 2016 I walked twelve kilometers in another charity event. My daily pain, however, remained the same and to some extent gradually became worse. I was healed; I knew this because I had had a number of MRI scans to show no more tissue damage. The pain continued and I found it hard to accept that I didn't need any more surgery. My brain was telling me otherwise and that was the truth that I listened to.

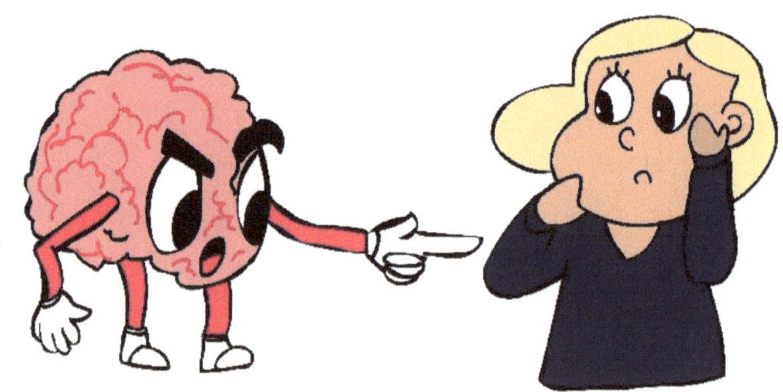

A dark place

After three years of constant, daily and nightly pain in my back and lower limbs, varying on a pain scale from 'three out of ten' to 'ten out of ten', and after two surgeries, numerous MRI scans, various concoctions of pain relief and almost two years of physiotherapy, I had reached the darkest, most scary part of my journey with persistent pain. This dark place was not a good place to be. It was something that found me in the early hours of the morning, most mornings, something that took me away from my family and friends and removed me, in my eyes, from the very face of useful and meaningful existence. With this came guilt, utter fear and a feeling of nowhere to go. I needed a diagnosis that would take away, remove, and permanently cut out my pain.

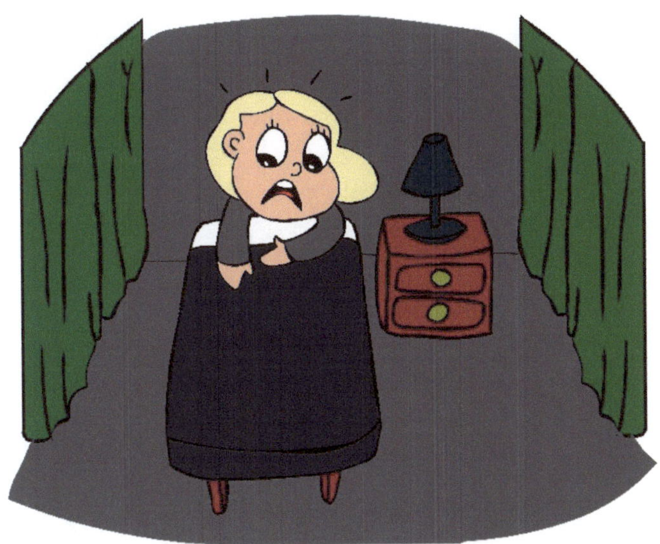

In March 2017 things were getting no better and my physiotherapy team suggested that I go on a pain contract, funded by the Accident Compensation Corporation, ACC. Although not too sure what this involved, I was desperate to give anything a go. Around the same time I had had my seventh MRI scan, which, of course, showed no real change in my physiology other than a small disc bulge and some scar tissue. More importantly, it meant that I needed to perhaps accept that something else was going on. Something that was maybe out of my control, that somehow my brain was possibly rewiring my nervous system to be more sensitive to pain than it should be.

I was diagnosed with chronic pain, but this was not the verdict I was looking for and, as far as I was concerned, it was not what I had. I didn't really understand what chronic pain was. Its very subject left me feeling uneasy, uncomfortable and a label used when all avenues had been exhausted, something that to me, and my lack of knowledge on the subject, meant that the pain was unlikely to go away. In my own mind, I felt that I was wasting the time of the health professionals who had worked so hard with me. I couldn't see how I would get through this, as I must have been imagining the pain, after all, the MRI showed no reason for me to be in this amount of discomfort.

Around this time, it was suggested that I read a book 'Explain Pain', by David S Butler and G Lorimer Mosely (Noigroup Publications, 2013). I was keen to open it up and consider that maybe I might have a new challenge ahead, an un-surgical route to getting well. Again, this didn't sit comfortably with me. The irony was that I was looking for a surgical approach to relieve me of the pain, but that very approach was the one thing that I dreaded the most and was petrified of. Go figure!

In the book I read about nociceptors, receptors in the neurons in our tissues that detect and alert us to danger. Apparently, nociception, when neurons in our tissues respond to danger, happens most of the time but it doesn't always end in pain. These neurons were sending **danger** messages to my spinal cord and brain. My brain was then analysing these messages as an indication of tissue danger. All this is well and good when you have real tissue damage. However, in my case, the nociceptors were giving me the **wrong** message, as I didn't have the tissue damage in my spine to warrant such alarming signals.

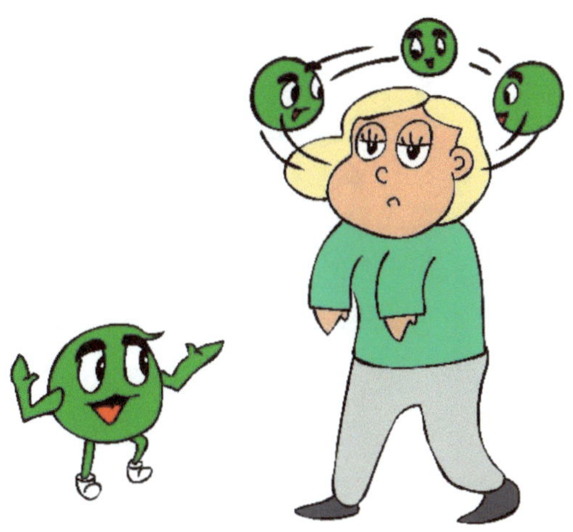

I like to use the word interceptor, instead of nociceptor, for the little voice in my head that suggests danger to me. Why the term interceptor you may ask? Well, what are interceptors? They are something that intercept or stop you from continuing on to a destination and that is what these brain messages were doing to me. They were stopping me from moving forward to my destination of pain free and happy living.

In my case, and I'm guessing that if you are reading this as a fellow chronic pain sufferer, you would most probably react the same way as I did with any increase in pain. The interceptors would send out a great big 'MAYDAY, MAYDAY, MAYDAY…listen to us, you need to act now, seek medical attention IMMEDIATELY!' I would react to this alert and look for all the cues that would tell me that I was in grave danger.

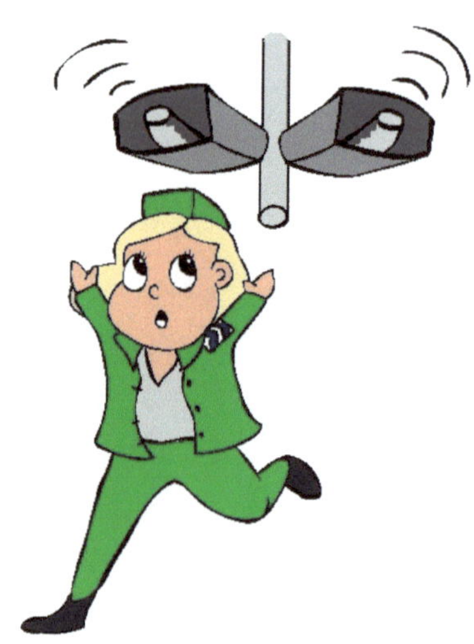

As a result, my entire mood would hit rock bottom and I would be totally convinced that surgery was necessary and no one would persuade me otherwise; after all, this is what had happened before, on two occasions, so why would it not be happening again?

Central Sensitisation

A meeting with a pain consultant was very reassuring. We looked together at the results of my eighth, yes, I'd had another one, MRI scan and once again I was told that surgery was not necessary. I was presented with images from the scan and they indicated that my spine was showing signs of degeneration. However, this level of degeneration was normal for my age. Apparently, many people have degenerative spinal conditions, far worse than mine and have no pain or idea of their level of degeneration. Interesting! Chronic pain with central sensitisation was diagnosed.

Reassurance that the pain was not in my head was not helpful. The pain was there, despite no deterioration on the MRI scans. This makes it very hard not to think you are going mad. At its worse my pain was 'eight out of ten' (**"Oh God, I think I am dying…I really need help."**) and at its best 'five out of ten' (**"No joking now, this is not funny!**). What was going on? Somehow, my brain had decided to over protect itself by sending out alarm bells, maydays and danger signals that I didn't need to act on.

So, not only chronic pain, but now something else on top - central sensitisation, which, in effect, maintains chronic pain. My interceptors were working overtime and in a persistent state of high alert. Things that normally didn't cause pain like light touch, were amplified and perceived as more painful. The pain was now becoming activated with thoughts, places, emotions and even pictures. This plays around with your thinking! How could something, such as a light touch, a memory or even an up-and-coming visit to a physiotherapist or doctor send a 'MAYDAY, MAYDAY, GET HELP, IMMEDIATELY' message to my brain?

The interceptors were saying "you need to get help, get the pain cut out, get advice, visit the doctor, have another MRI" (which would be sure to show a massive, bulging, herniated disc the size of Gibraltar), "stay off work, don't lift, don't bend, don't exercise" and importantly "don't accept that this is not real damage that doesn't need immediate surgery".

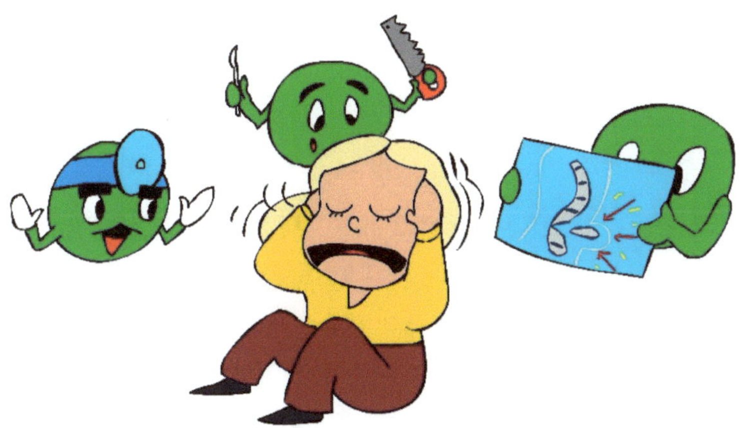

Flare-ups

Early in June 2017, I was admitted to hospital with suspected viral meningitis. To confirm the diagnosis, a lumber puncture was carried out in order to collect a sample of cerebrospinal fluid. This procedure proved to be quite difficult to complete due to my previous two spinal surgeries and scar tissue in the lumbar spine area. As a result, I ended up with a post-lumber puncture headache, on top of all the other pain I was experiencing.

A post-lumber puncture headache is a common occurrence and happens in ten to thirty percent of patients after a lumber puncture. As a result, I spent the best part of three weeks lying horizontal in bed. I don't quite know whether the needle used in the lumber puncture, or the horizontal position that I had to endure while my headache went away, aggravated the back pain but bang! A flare-up! Oh my, had I endured a few of those? Another couple of words that I didn't like and a grey area I felt. A flare-up can mean a few things; no cause for concern, the result of increased activity, irritation to an old injury, or new pain that needs medical attention.

When I experienced a flare-up, caused by one of many possibilities, I waited patiently for the red flag symptoms to show. For me red flag symptoms were a pre-curser to Cauda Equina Syndrome (CES), something that I narrowly avoided after my initial injury went badly wrong. Symptoms include low back pain, pain that radiates down both legs, numbness around the area that would normally sit in a saddle, and loss of bowel or bladder control. Over time, my symptoms didn't become any worse. However, for someone with chronic pain and an experience of a very scary painful episode, you sit like a frightened possum in a headlight, waiting for it all to go wrong. Because it will, won't it? It did before and it will again. Is that not the case?

To me, it really didn't matter how many times I was told that, "we've been here before, you got over this last time" or "you were doing so well before". A new flare-up meant a new certainty that things had gone badly wrong again. When experiencing a flare-up I would feel helpless, sad, worried and get myself back into that dark space again.

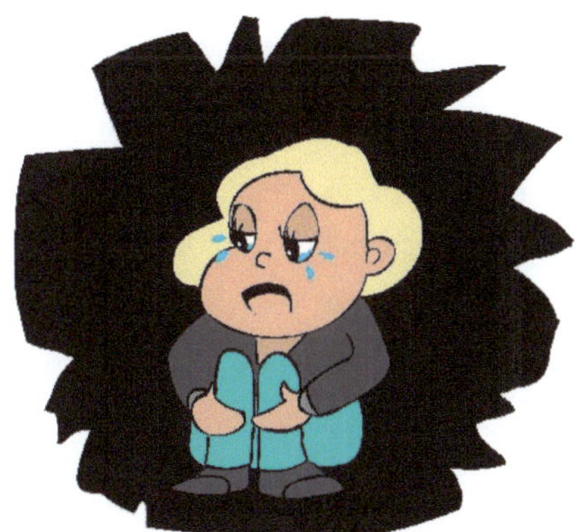

Gradually my flare-ups began to get worse and the pain would no longer be isolated to my back and lower legs. I would ache in just about every joint in my body. I would struggle to stand, sit, lie down, sleep, walk and even bend my fingers. When this happened I would be in my most miserable place. I wondered about carrying on. I was over the pain, the visits to the doctor, the promises that things would get better, the soul destroying times when I was doing well and then bang, back to square one again. More importantly, I was becoming embarrassed about talking about my condition. People expect you to get better, they expect you to heal. So, when you don't…

During a flare-up the nerve pain in my legs would worsen. I can only really describe the pain as an intense burning that occurred in any part of my right and sometimes left leg. It was a little like having a lit match held in one spot for about two seconds and utter agony. The pain could happen in one toe, my knee, my butt cheek or in any number of places in my lower extremity. In addition, I would not sleep at night and would wake up with excruciating leg cramps or back spasms. Under these circumstances, trying not to think the worse was not easy. For me I was so afraid of getting back to that 'eleven out of ten' pain that anything reminding me of that episode made me feel helpless, out of control, and more importantly very frightened.

I'd try anything I could to relieve the pain, from heat, movement, socialising, talking about it, to not talking about it, rest, pain relief and sleep, the latter to blot out the pain. I didn't know what else to do.

I felt sorry for my family and friends, my health professionals and anyone who had been helping me to find the Holy Grail of cures and remedies. I wasn't terminally ill. I had the rest of my life to look forward to. I should be grateful, not depressed, and certainly not thinking about throwing in the towel. I knew that I needed to do one of two things, either carry on in this state of helplessness, that may have led to who knows what, or take some new ideas on board and believe in them.

Back to happiness

As part of the pain contract package, funded by ACC, I had access to one-on-one consultations with a pain psychologist. I was initially a little reluctant to go down this road, as I didn't really want to accept that I had a mental health issue. However, I knew now that the pain was getting out of *my* control and this was terrifying. It was time for me to move forward. The little voices in my head, the interceptors, were reminding me of past pain experiences. ***Point to note, pain messages are useful in most cases, but with me they had become harmful.*** They were mentally harming me and the usual solution, of my reaction to the pain, had become the problem.

After a few consultations with my pain psychologist I began to realise that I was not accepting the pain for what it was. I was hanging on to old pain memories and was either acting on them and rushing to get medical help, or ignoring them and trying to push them to the back of my mind. Both approaches were ineffective and led to a vicious cycle of unhappiness and increased pain.

Worse still, I was beginning to feel upset and angry with myself for allowing the second injury to happen. I blamed myself for being stupid enough to have followed the doctor's instruction to bend down after my first surgery. I was looking for blame and I felt hurt, let down and helpless.

At this time, my pain psychologist recommended another book to me, 'The Happiness Trap' by Russ Harris (Little Brown Book

Group Publications). This book is centered on Mindfulness, Acceptance, and Commitment Therapy (ACT) and is well worth a read. Reading the book led me to a new realisation that I had to commit to accepting the pain for what it *really* was. It helped me to understand that thoughts about pain can be either *helpful* or *unhelpful*. The thoughts I had, in relation to my persistent pain, were *unhelpful*, they alerted me to the *wrong* responses and didn't give me the correct information about what was going on in my tissues.

I needed to step back, ACT technique, from my thoughts and see them for what they really were. I needed to diffuse them. There are many techniques for doing this and you would have to read the book and work through the exercises yourself to do this.

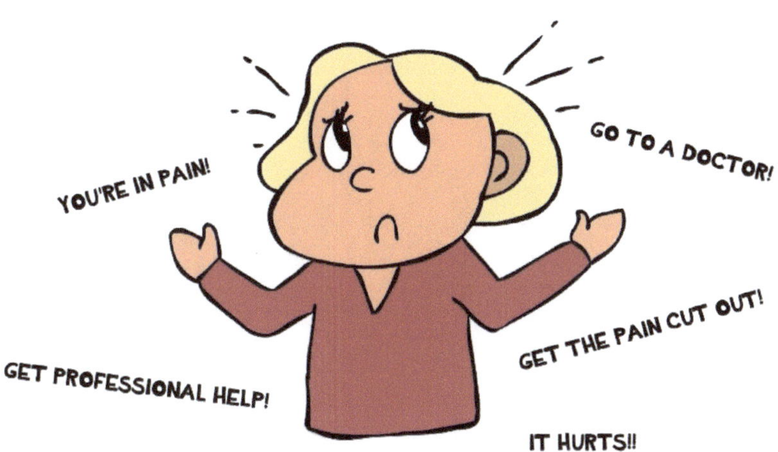

With ACT you learn that negative thoughts are only a problem if you act on them and give them your full attention. Instead, you acknowledge the thought, in my case the painful thought, and let it be. Don't give it much attention, let it pass and channel your energy into doing something else more worthwhile, in other words, distract yourself. With chronic pain, this only works if you accept the fact that you have **no** tissue damage and **no** reason for your 'interceptors' to be alerting you to danger. You have to completely commit to this technique, otherwise it **will not** work.

I really recommend both books, 'Explain Pain' and 'The Happiness Trap'. Together they helped me change my thinking about the pain I was experiencing and how to finally start moving forward.

A new diet

About the time I had started to practice my ACT techniques, I happened to be lying on the couch surfing Netflix for something to watch. I came across a documentary about diet and how this can have a huge effect on health. Heaven knows we have been inundated with wonderful diets and cures, from cutting out fat, adding in fat, eating meat, not eating meat, eating no carbs, eating all carbs, cutting out sugar...the list is endless. Anyway, I watched and learnt about detoxing with a diet of fruit and vegetable juice. Amazing things seemed to have happened to people who initially fasted on this diet and then made it a major part of their daily food intake. Lo and behold, a woman talked about her disc problem and bi-lateral leg pain and how this had disappeared. That's when my ears pricked up and I started to take notice.

It seems that we hale from an age where we ate mainly fruit and plant food with the odd animal thrown in here and there - when we could catch one of course. Therefore, we really had a few choices in our diet, fruits and vegetables or meat, only the meat was not always available.

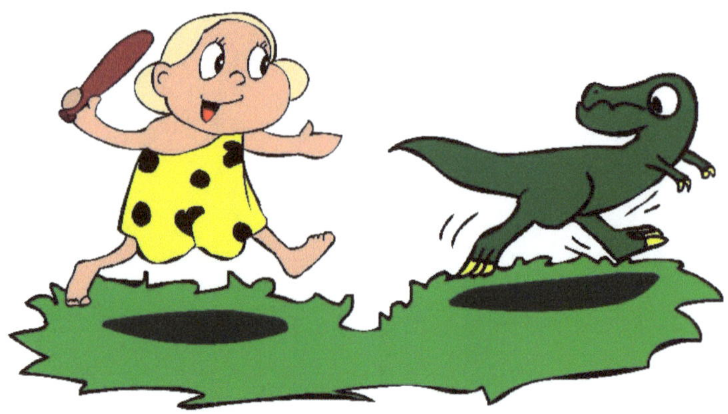

Nowadays we have an additional category to choose from, processed food. With our busy schedules and other excuses, a large proportion of us have changed our diet to eating mainly from this latter category, with a bit of meat and very little fruit and vegetables thrown in. "We have heard this all before", I'm sure you are shouting. Yes, and so had I, but this time it seemed to make sense. Many of us have cut out our natural antihistamines, anti-inflammatories and a whole heap of other good stuff that we need in our diet. Stuff that stops us from getting sick and heals us when we are in pain.

So, ready to give anything a try, I began the next quest to support my journey of 'pain-freeness' with a diet of fruit and vegetable juice. At the time, I was at the beginning of a three-week holiday from work and I thought that this would be the ideal opportunity to get into a routine and see if it would make any difference. In my reckoning, twenty one days should have given me an indication of whether this was going to make a difference or not.

A diet of just fruit and vegetable juice didn't really suit me, as I like physical food to chew on. So instead, I cut out all white sugar, white flour, potatoes, white rice, pasta and red meat, eating mainly fruit, green vegetables, nuts, wholegrains, chicken and oily fish. By day three, I recorded a 'two out of ten' on two occasions in my pain diary. I couldn't remember the last time I had had a score so low.

My initial euphoria was replaced with a little skepticism as the numbers steadily rose to 'five out of ten'. However, by day four I was averaging 'four to five' out of ten with bottom scores of 'three out of ten'. Compared with a previous long-term average days of 'six to seven out of ten', things were definitely looking better. I was particularly pleased with myself when on day five I went ice-skating with my grandson. Despite the voices in my head and from my husband, saying "no, don't do it", I did it. And… no after affects, no falls, no pain, WOW!

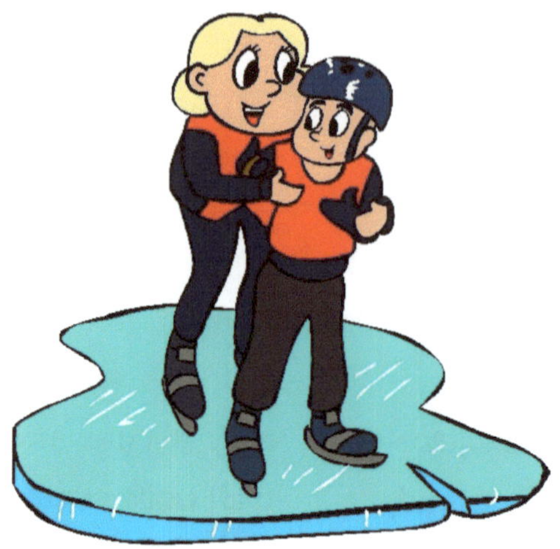

Day seven looked very promising with 'three out of ten' being my average recorded number and only 'five out of ten' recorded twice. The main thing was that the intense pain I normally had at night was changing. More importantly, the nerve pain was almost non-existent with only a couple of episodes per day, compared to hundreds. I still had the back pain at night but somehow it seemed different. Keeping my numbers below 'five out of ten' now became my goal. My first night of being almost pain free happened on day eight.

I decided to do a little research on foods naturally containing anti-inflammatories. These food groups include tomatoes, olive oil, green leafy vegetables, apples, whole grains, nuts such as almonds and walnuts, fatty fish such as salmon, mackerel, tuna and sardines, and fruit such as strawberries, blueberries, cherries and oranges. In addition, these food groups reduce the risk of

chronic diseases and overall improve mood and quality of life. More importantly, I noted the foods that I usually ate, refined carbs, such as white bread and pastries, French fries and other fried food, sugars, especially chocolate, red meats, sausage and margarine, inflame and accelerate the inflammatory process.

My next finding was spirulina, a bluey green looking powder, which is a natural algae high in protein with a good source of nutrients, vitamin B and antioxidants; it seemingly has a whole wealth of health benefits. Apparently, one teaspoon of this a day gives your body a natural energy boost, note to self, take in the morning not before bed, as it helps improve the immune system, supports the heart, liver and kidneys and is a natural detoxifier, cleansing the body of toxins. More importantly to me it seems to help balance the body's pH, reducing inflammation in a safe and chemical-free way. So, one teaspoon of this per day was added to my diet.

Gradually, I was getting my pain under control and because of this I was able to exercise and get out-and-about again. My pain scale gradually reduced and averaged 'three to four out of ten'. I recorded my first full night's sleep within a month of using my new ACT techniques and changed diet. Some days I even recorded a zero for a large part of the day.

From zero to ten and back again

Not too long after the pain had started to settle I experienced my first major flare-up and was woken up with a 'MAYDAY, MAYDAY, WAKE UP, WE'RE IN TROUBLE' from my interceptors.

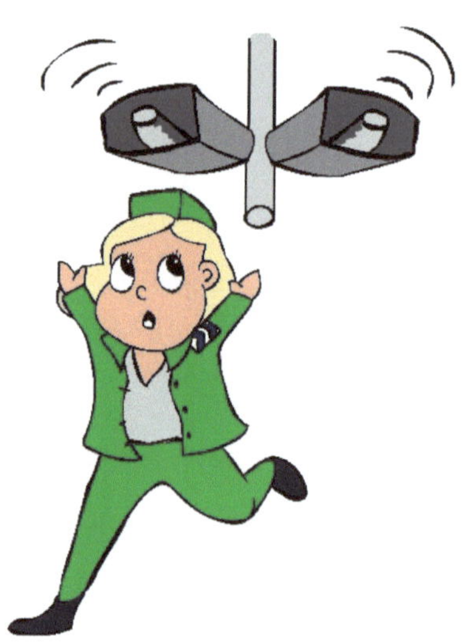

I was quite surprised at the level of high alert that my body was in, especially since I had almost got on top of all this pain now. I had had a few pain free days and was beginning to tell people that I was cured. I remembered my pain psychologist saying that chronic pain does have a tendency to flare-up, but I didn't expect it to happen quite this soon. I analysed the reason for the flare-up. I had had a busy week at work and some emotional altercations had played on my mind. I identified that these were the triggers since I hadn't fallen, twisted, lifted or done anything to harm my back. Identifying triggers for a flare-up is the most important thing to getting on top of them. This, for me, was an important lesson to learn.

This flare-up was the most frightening to date. I woke up and struggled to stand because of the nerve pain in my feet. Every bone in my body ached. My knees were so sore that I couldn't walk. My fingers were swollen and I couldn't open my hands. I felt sick to my stomach and was an emotional wreck. The pain was no longer isolated to my back and right leg, it had risen to a completely new level. I was tempted to go to the doctor, to email my pain team, but instead, I put my ACT Therapy into action and didn't give the pain the attention it craved. I had had a taster of 'pain freeness' and this was where I was heading. I decided to be brave and hit this flare-up full on.

First of all I acknowledged the pain for what it was, a flare-up and just a flare-up. I acknowledged and accepted that the pain was nothing to worry about. I didn't take any medication but instead made myself quite busy. Distraction, not ignoring, is important here. I was aware of the pain, but just defused the interceptors as best as I could by keeping myself busy.

I did everything from emptying the dishwasher, which was very difficult to do since my hands and fingers were stiff, to putting a load of washing in the washing machine, making breakfast. I got myself showered and dressed and drove to town to post a letter, crying all the way home as the pain was so bad. I couldn't imagine the pain going by itself and was very tempted to take medication. Throughout the day I recorded pain scores from 'eight out of ten' on the pain scale to 'five out of ten' by bed time.

The following day I was still in some discomfort but continued to distract myself. By the end of the second day the pain was down to 'three out of ten' and by the third day I was back to zero.

If you have ever watched the movie, 'The Awakenings' (a 1990 American drama based on Oliver Sacks's memoir) a flare-up feels a little like that. Coming out of a dark place into the light and then, bang, back into the dark again. A cruel experience that we, as chronic pain sufferers, face. It was after this major flare-up that I realised that my journey with chronic pain was not going to be easy. I wasn't cured as I thought, just temporarily relieved. I knew now that I wouldn't be able to predict a flare-up, I also knew that I wouldn't be able to predict how long I would be pain free. More importantly though, I now had some strategies to put in place when things went wrong. I guess an analogy would be people living with epilepsy, diabetes, arthritis and-so-on. These are conditions, without a cure, that people learn to live with but have tools to deal with their disorder. The tools could be medication, mindfulness, psychology, physiotherapy, diet etc. and for us, dear fellow chronic pain sufferers, we have to do the same. Accept the pain for what it is and deal with it. Get our tools out of the toolbox and learn to live again.

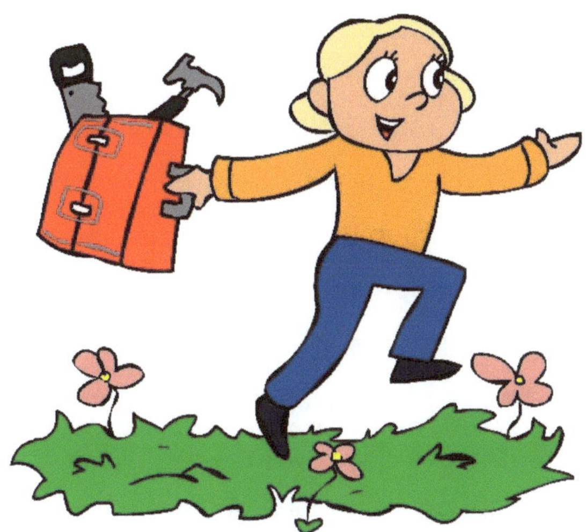

Adjustment to life

Throughout the three-and-a-half years of my recovery from surgeries and having to deal with living with chronic pain, I always maintained a determination to return to work. Initially this was not possible and I had seven months off work. Whether it's me, being an active relaxer, or just that I get bored easy, I don't know. Nonetheless, I always made a determined effort to return to work. Believe me, this was never an easy choice. It began with me working for just a couple of hours a day and having to have taxi rides and colleagues drive me to work. This went on for about six months.

I gradually increased my working hours until I was able to complete a full day. Next, I had to find ways of driving to and from work comfortably and safely. I had a back support in the car to help, and I eventually changed my car to one that had a reversing camera and cruise control. This was the only way I could drive long distances and avoid leg spasms, as keeping my leg straight for any great length of time was painful. Also turning around to reverse was not good.

As chronic pain sufferers, I'm afraid we have to adjust our lives. For me, I never drive forward into a supermarket space now unless I can also drive forwards out of it. Sometimes it means waiting for a space, but so be it.

For a few reasons I never use a big deep supermarket trolley for my grocery shopping any more. Firstly, I shop little and often and use the smaller less deep trolleys and, when at home and away from work and people, it means you have to get out more often into the 'real world' making you feel happier as you socialise. Secondly, bending down to put items in and then take items out of a deep trolley, just aggravates things. Thirdly, a smaller amount of shopping is easier to get into the house when you get home.

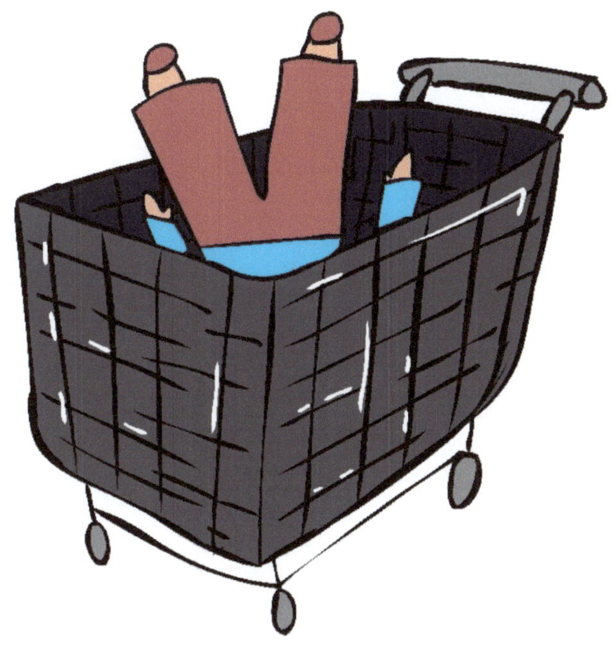

Persistent pain becomes a real problem when you give in to it. You may not feel that you are giving in to the pain, however, if because of it, you are not working, struggling with relationships and feeling depressed, then I'm afraid you are, as I most definitely was. Remember, chronic pain does ***not*** mean real tissue damage, once you accept that, then you can start your journey towards a happier and more meaningful life.

Don't underestimate the help from your health professionals

I've mentioned physiotherapists, psychologists, doctors, surgeons and dieticians who all, as a team, work together to get you back on your feet. One other important member of the rehabilitation team is the occupational therapist. These wonderful people come into hospital; visit you in your own home and workplace. They help patients improve their skills for day-to-day activities and well-being. I was provided with a number of devices to help me recuperate. These included push-along trollies, for hanging out my washing and as a food cart, a Reacher and Grabber to pick things up when I struggled to bend, a shower seat, a portable grab handle to help me get in and out of the bath, footwear to help me with walking as I trained, a back support for the car and a whole lot of other helpful, useful items that made my recovery so much easier. Probably my saving grace was an adjustable height desk and chair which made my return to work possible and to which I still rely on to this day.

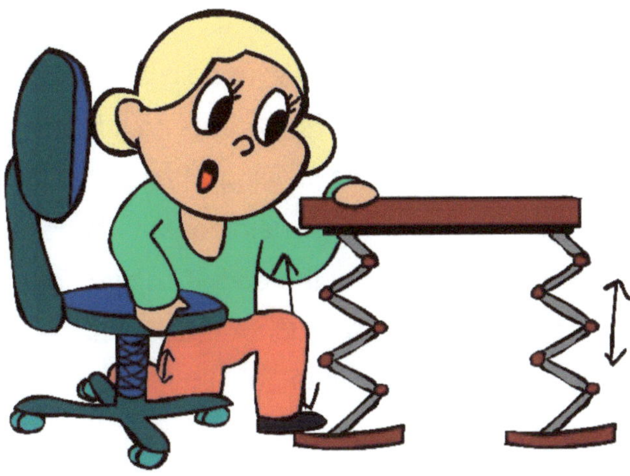

It's up to you to move forward

I continue to live with the unpredictable condition of chronic pain. Every day is different and as I climb out of bed I never know what each day will bring. Some days and weeks I feel amazing and others not so. I know what it is like to be at rock bottom, I know how it feels to worry that relationships, friendships, finances etc. may be jeopardised because of this disorder. You are never alone as millions of people of all ages and from all over the world suffer from some form of chronic pain.

Everyone's experience with persistent pain is different and unique and there is no 'one remedy fits all' solution. This story has been my account of the journey I have had with chronic pain and how I came to accept and deal with it. I cannot truthfully say that any one solution was better than the other when it came to reducing my pain score. It was the holistic collaboration of doctors, physiotherapists, psychotherapists, occupational health workers and a change in diet, exercise and thinking that collectively contributed to my well-being.

Finally, never have any doubt that your pain isn't real. However, know that you can move forward by accepting it for what it has become and take the first steps to living with pain and having a happier and healthier life. Chronic pain does not mean the end of happiness and it certainly is not the end of enjoyment of life. I wake every morning and thank God for the life I have as things could have been very different if I had let this beast beat me. Join me on the journey to happiness.

Endnote

"For a long time it seemed to me that life was about to begin-real life. But there was always some obstacle in the way; something to be gotten through first, some unfinished business, time still to be served, a debt to be paid. At last it dawned on me that these obstacles were my life. This perspective has helped me to see that there is no way to happiness. Happiness is the way. So treasure every moment you have and remember that time waits for no one...Happiness is a journey...not a destination" (Alfred D. Souza).

ABOUT THE AUTHOR

Although now living in Te Awamutu, New Zealand, Michelle was born and raised in Conisborough, a small village near Doncaster, South Yorkshire, England. Michelle is married with two daughters, a grandson and a granddaughter and works as Head of Music at a secondary school in the Waikato region.